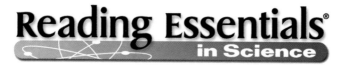

Reading Essentials®
in Science

HEALTHY LIVING

Alcohol, Tobacco, and Drugs

ALEXANDRA POWE ALLRED

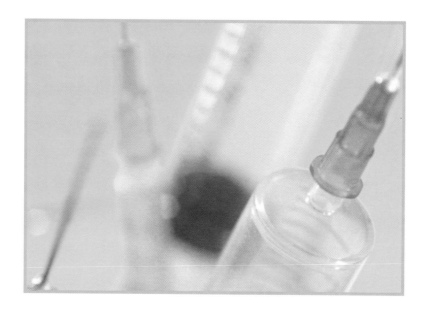

PERFECTION LEARNING®

Editorial Director: Susan C. Thies
Editor: Paula J. Reece
Design Director: Randy Messer
Book Design: Emily J. Greazel
Cover Design: Michael A. Aspengren

Thank you to my mother and father who taught me how to live a healthy life and be the happy person I am today. Your love is the best medicine!

Image credits:

© Brand X: p. 14 (right); © Zuma Press/ZUMA/CORBIS: p. 9; © Hulton-Deutsch Collection/ CORBIS: p. 11; © Lester V. Bergman/CORBIS: p. 13 (right), © Joel W. Rogers/CORBIS: p. 15 (bottom); © Scott Houston/CORBIS: p. 20; © Associated Press: p. 26

Argosy Illustration: p. 13 (left); Banana Stock Royalty Free: p. 33; ClipArt.com: pp. 15 (top), 22, 23; Creatas Royalty Free: p. 35; Image 100: pp. 3, 16; LifeArt © 2003 Lippincott, Williams, & Wilkins: pp. 6, 8; Map Resources: p. 14 (bottom); Pefection Learning: pp. 19, 21; PhotoDisc Royalty Free: p. 30; Photos.com: back cover, front cover, pp. 4, 5, 7, 12, 17, 24, 27, 28

A special thanks to the following for her scientific review of the book:

Dr. Marcie R. Wycoff-Horn, Assistant Professor, Department of Health Education and Health Promotion, University of Wisconsin-LaCrosse

1 2 3 4 5 6 PP 09 08 07 06 05 04

ISBN 0-7891-6441-8

Table of Contents

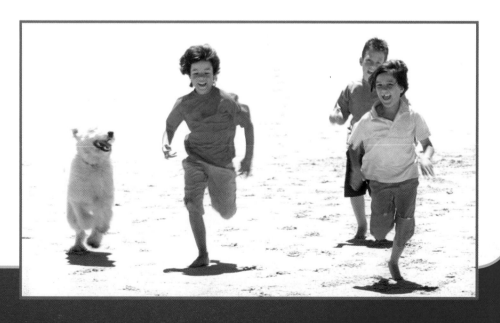

Introduction to Alcohol, Tobacco, and Drugs

Every day, you put things into your body. Food, water, and the air you breathe are all necessary for you to live and be healthy. But there are many things people put into their bodies that are harmful. These things don't help you

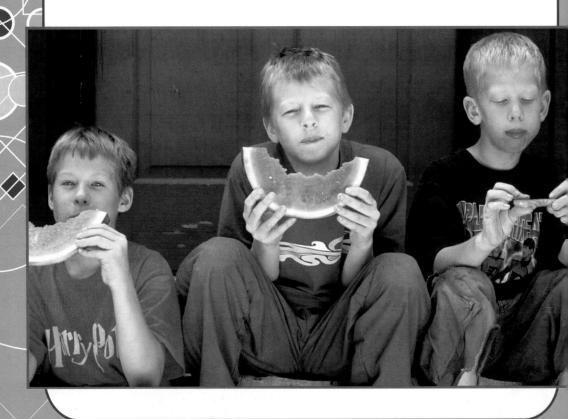

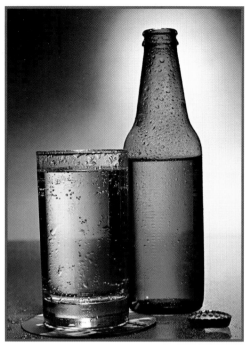

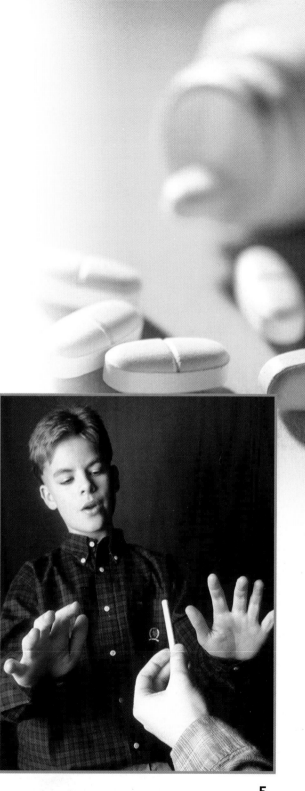

grow bigger, stronger, and smarter. Instead, they mess with your brain, cause diseases—and can even kill you.

Alcohol, **tobacco**, and **drugs** are all harmful to your body. However, many kids (and adults) use and abuse these substances. Nearly every kid is tempted to try alcohol, tobacco, or drugs at some time. But learning what these poisons can do to you will give you more reasons to say no.

Down the Drain
Alcohol and Your Body

You have probably seen a cartoon in which a mouse or cat falls into a barrel of alcohol. The next thing you know, the silly animal has the hiccups and is walking around doing funny things. The truth is, alcohol is not that funny.

What Is Alcohol?

Alcohol is a drug. A drug is a chemical that changes the way your body works. Alcohol is a **depressant** that slows down your brain, making you feel more relaxed. But it does more than just relax your brain. It kills brain cells. That's what's happening when people who are drinking lose their balance, have difficulty speaking, and do foolish things.

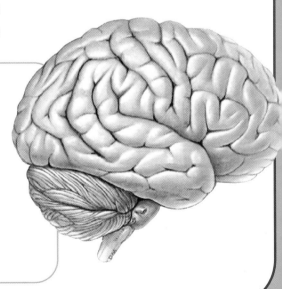

What Are Brain Cells?

You were born with a certain number of brain cells. Your brain cells make connections with one another. These connections make you able to learn. When your brain cells die (or you kill them by drinking alcohol), they are not replaced.

If you drink too much, you become **intoxicated**, or drunk. This may cause you to become sick and vomit or even pass out or become unconscious. But the problems don't end once you've woken up. When you wake up, you will likely have a **hangover**. You will have a horrible headache and a very upset stomach. You may even vomit again. This lasts for hours. Unfortunately, when children and teenagers drink, most drink in order to get drunk. Imagine *choosing* to feel sick!

Drinking too much in a short time can give you more than a headache. It can actually kill you. This is called *alcohol poisoning*. It may start with **vomiting**. Your brain signals your stomach to get rid of the alcohol because it detects that there is too much in your body. Vomiting is your body's way of getting rid of the poison.

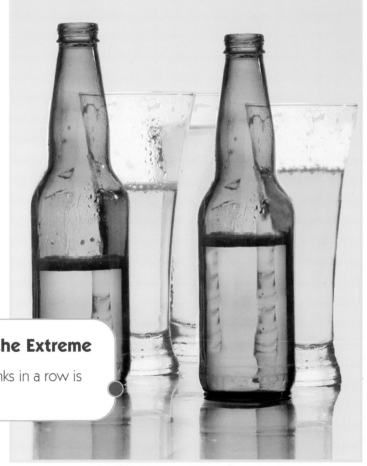

If you have drunk a **lethal** amount of alcohol, your body will start to shut down. Remember how alcohol is a depressant? Well, if you drink too much, it can depress, or relax, your **central nervous system** too much. That means the alcohol can shut off the areas of your brain that control **consciousness**, breathing, and heart rate. What happens then? You fall into a **coma**. If you don't get help in time, you die. Your friends may think you have just passed out. But in reality, you may never wake up.

Another way alcohol poisoning can kill you is when you've already passed out and your brain tells your stomach to make you vomit. If you are too drunk to wake up and clear out your airway, you will choke on the vomit and die. You may hear friends or older kids say, "Drinking is so fun!" Does this sound fun to you?

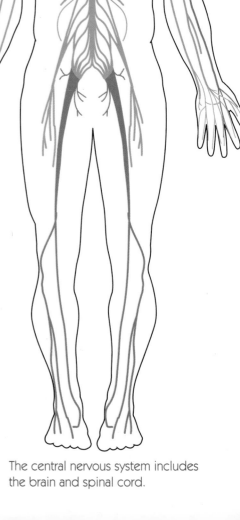

The central nervous system includes the brain and spinal cord.

Alcohol Poisoning—What to Look For

The signs of alcohol poisoning are:
- vomiting
- passing out
- difficulty awakening
- breathing slowly and shallowly

There are many reasons young people should not drink. Alcohol slows down the healthy development of muscles and bones. If you drink while you are still growing and developing, you may be smaller than other kids. Alcohol makes it harder to fight off diseases because it weakens your **immune system**. That means you are more likely to get sick. Studies also show that if you start young, you are more likely to become hooked. Kids who start drinking before age 15 are four times more likely to become **alcoholics** than their friends who don't drink.

What Is an Alcoholic?

Alcoholics are people who constantly crave alcohol. They are **addicted**. Even though alcohol is bad for them, their brain begins to play tricks on them, sending the message that alcohol is a good thing. Alcoholics are unable to stop drinking without help. Because alcoholism is a disease, it does not go away. Recovering alcoholics are people who, with help, have been able to stop drinking. However, they know that they must never drink alcohol again.

Alcohol Can Kill

Alcohol is involved in the three leading causes of teen deaths—automobile crashes, homicides, and suicides.

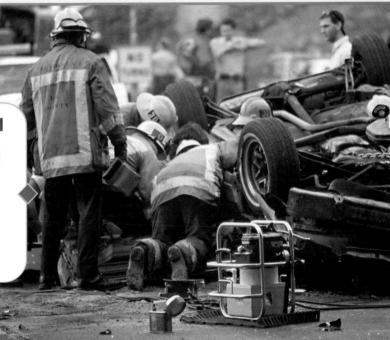

Just because your mother, father, grandparent, or guardian drinks a beer or a glass of wine, however, does not mean he or she is an alcoholic. There is a reason that alcohol consumption is legal for adults 21 and older. Since kids' and teenagers' bodies are still developing, alcohol has a much greater impact on them. Their health is affected more. Adults are more likely to have the maturity and experience to make responsible decisions when it comes to drinking.

Alcoholism—Know the Signs

Below are signs that someone you care about may have a drinking problem:

- Having more than a couple drinks a day for a series of days
- Lying about how much he or she has had to drink
- Making excuses for needing a drink
- Drinking alone or hiding his or her drinking
- Forgetting things or breaking promises
- Choosing drinking over other activities he or she once enjoyed

You may be thinking, "But how can I say no? Everyone's doing it—right?" *Wrong*. Movies and television shows make drinking alcohol look like a lot of fun. T.V. commercials for beer products show parties with people singing, dancing, laughing, and drinking beer. All the people look attractive and cool. But it is important to remember that the advertisements are misleading. It may seem like everyone's doing it. Especially if your friends are pressuring you to go drinking. But in reality, most kids and teenagers *don't* drink alcohol. Research shows that 70 percent of people ages 12 to 20 haven't drunk alcohol in the past month. That's way over half! It's tough to say no. You want to be popular. You want to appear cool. But if you say no, you're actually in the majority. Not only that, you'll be saying yes to good health—and to life.

People ages 12 to 20 who haven't drunk alcohol in the past month

Up in Smoke
The Truth About Tobacco

Early Americans learned how to smoke loose leaves of tobacco in long pipes. By the 19th century, Europeans and Americans learned to roll shredded tobacco in thin strips of paper, calling them **cigarettes**. During World War I, free cigarettes were given to U.S. soldiers so they could "relax" on breaks from the fighting. By the time World War I ended, thousands of Americans who had never smoked were introduced to cigarettes. Many were addicted by the time they returned home. Soldiers were not the only ones suddenly interested in the cigarettes. When women were given the right to vote in 1920, many took up smoking as well. Like voting, smoking had long been something only men could do. So many women believed smoking was a symbol of their new independence. Of course, this was before scientists and doctors learned how harmful the tobacco plant is.

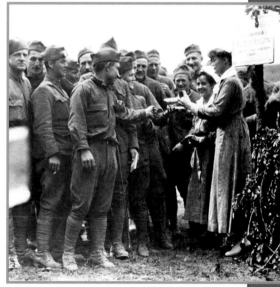

The American Red Cross distributed cigarettes to soldiers during World War I.

Tobacco is a plant with long, broad leaves and pink or red flowers. The plant doesn't look dangerous, but it can be a killer. Tobacco can be smoked in cigarettes, pipes, or cigars. It can also be placed between the gums and sucked on. This is called **smokeless tobacco.**

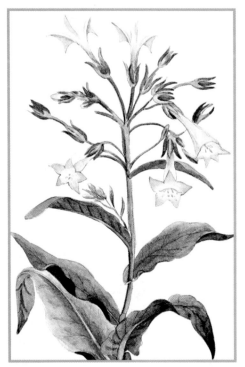

Tobacco plant

One reason tobacco is so harmful is because it contains **nicotine**. This is a chemical that makes you feel good for a short time. However, nicotine is also extremely addictive. You can become seriously hooked even days after you first "experiment" with smoking. And addiction to smoking can lead to serious health problems and even death. Today, tobacco use kills more people than **AIDS**, alcohol, drug abuse, car crashes, murders, and suicides—all combined! Each year more than 430,000 people die from using tobacco.

What Smoking Does to the Body

Smoking makes it harder for you to breathe. When you breathe, your **lungs** convert air into **oxygen** and other gases that your body needs to survive. Those gases then enter your blood. That's why it is so important for you to breathe clean, fresh air. You wouldn't want to wash your clothing in muddy water or put garbage instead of gasoline into your family car's fuel line. But when you use tobacco, the chemicals and ingredients are also carried into your bloodstream. Each time you puff on a cigarette, you are putting poison into your body.

Your body works hard to clean the bad air from your body. Each time you breathe out, you exhale **carbon dioxide**—a waste product—from your lungs. This is important, as your body needs to get rid of the carbon dioxide and keep your body clean. Inside your lungs are little air sacs called *alveoli*, which are found at the end of the **bronchial tubes**. It is important to keep those air sacs clean so you can take deep, healthy breaths of air. Think of your bronchial tubes and lungs as a kitchen sink. Imagine if every time you cleaned the dishes after dinner, you put all the leftover food down the kitchen sink drain but never ran the garbage disposal. Eventually, the sink would get clogged up and begin to overflow onto the kitchen floor. When you smoke, you are clogging up your air sacs with a nasty, tarlike substance. You find it harder to run and think. Even worse, smoking can cause diseases in your lungs and heart. If these organs become too damaged, you can die. Smoking also causes **cancer**. In fact, there are 40 different chemicals in tobacco smoke that are known to cause cancer.

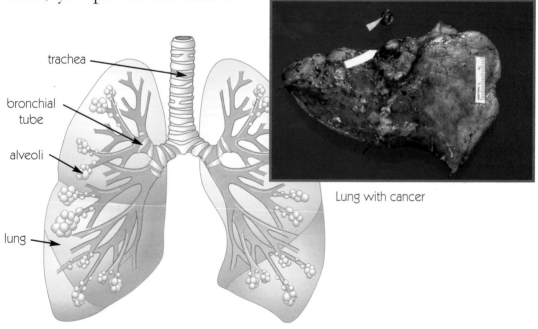

Lung with cancer

trachea

bronchial tube

alveoli

lung

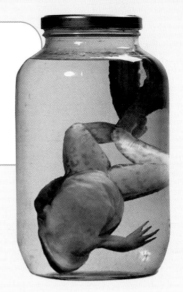

No Butts About It— Kids Shouldn't Smoke

Young people are especially at risk from smoking. Even though some of the effects of smoking, like cancer, don't show up right away, some symptoms can start with your first cigarette. The **surgeon general** reports that wheezing and coughing have been found in kids who smoke just one cigarette a week.

Kids are also more likely to get hooked than adults. More than one-third of all kids who ever smoke a cigarette become daily smokers before leaving high school.

Tobacco companies are counting on this. Think about it: Almost 90 percent of adults who smoke began at or before age 18. So the success of tobacco companies depends on you and your friends! Without kids who smoke, tobacco companies wouldn't have a future. The tobacco companies have faced many lawsuits about how they **market** their products. Some documents that have been brought out during the lawsuits

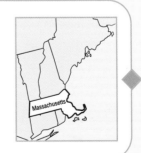

show that companies have targeted kids as young as 13 as a key market. They studied the smoking habits of kids so they could make products and advertising aimed directly at them.

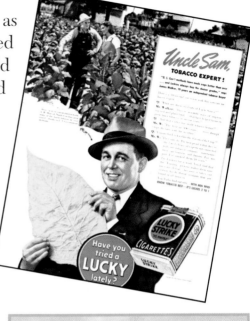

And advertising seems to lure kids more than adults to buy certain tobacco products. Only half of adult smokers buy the three most heavily advertised brands of cigarettes. However, 85 percent of kids ages 12 to 17 choose these brands. Cigarette companies claim that they have stopped targeting kids. But some people feel that the companies are finding other ways to get to kids. Their wallets depend on you!

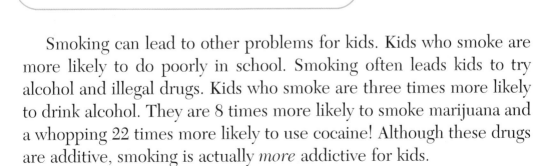

Joe Seemed Cool to Kids

Between 1989 and 1993, spending on the Joe Camel campaign for one tobacco company increased from $27 million to $43 million. This increase in advertising had no effect on sales to adult smokers. But what about kids? The sales to youth smokers went up 50 percent!

Smoking can lead to other problems for kids. Kids who smoke are more likely to do poorly in school. Smoking often leads kids to try alcohol and illegal drugs. Kids who smoke are three times more likely to drink alcohol. They are 8 times more likely to smoke marijuana and a whopping 22 times more likely to use cocaine! Although these drugs are additive, smoking is actually *more* addictive for kids.

The good news is that although 4,000 kids try smoking for the first time each day, that doesn't mean "everyone's doing it." According to the surgeon general, only 13 percent of kids have smoked in the past 30 days. Of these, only 8 percent are regular smokers. So most kids aren't smoking. And if you stay smoke-free throughout school, you probably won't ever smoke! Take a deep breath, and enjoy a healthy life!

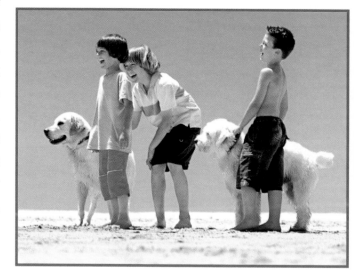

Try This!

The average daily smoker smokes 18 cigarettes per day. A pack contains 20 cigarettes, so that means the average smoker smokes .9 of a pack a day.

The average pack of cigarettes in the nation costs $3.81. So, to figure out how much the average smoker spends per day, multiply $3.81 by .9.

$$\begin{array}{r} 3.81 \\ \times \quad .9 \\ \hline \end{array}$$

How much, then, does the average smoker spend each year on cigarettes? To figure this, take the amount spent per day and multiply that by the number of days in a year.

Once you've figured out how much the average smoker spends each year on cigarettes, think about that cost. What could you buy or do with that money? With a partner, brainstorm what that money could buy, such as video games, new clothes, or books. You could even figure out how much money you could save if you put that money away for five or ten years. If you really want a challenge, figure how much money you could save if you put it in a savings account that pays interest! Make a poster that shows what a year's worth of smoking can buy.

Drugs: The Good, the Bad, and the Ugly

Humans have been using drugs in one form or another for hundreds and thousands of years. Natural **herbs**, trees, and roots have been used to treat headaches, fevers, and stomach pains. When early pioneers came to America, they brought many herbs from Europe with them, unsure of what they would find in the new land. They planted the herbs and made their own medicines. They also learned from Native Americans who taught them how to treat different illnesses and injuries with local herbs.

As the settlers learned more about how to use natural herbs, they were able to create powders for pills to fight infections and diseases, treat nerves with teas, and make lotions to soothe rashes and burns. Many of those very herbs are still found in lotions, vitamins, and drugs today.

Take Some Tree Bark and Call Me in the Morning

Native Americans figured out that chewing the inside bark of a willow tree worked as a pain reliever. Today, the aspirin in your medicine cabinet is made from this substance.

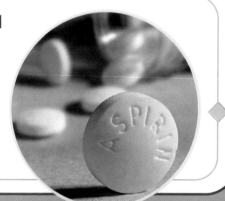

Today, some drugs are produced from plants or chemicals manufactured in laboratories. Among these are **prescription drugs**. These are the medicines that doctors give you when you are sick. Prescription drugs are ordered by a doctor from a pharmacy. They come with very specific directions about how to take them. You have probably seen your mother, father, or guardian read directions before giving you liquid medication or a pill. That is because your age, weight, or the illness you have makes a difference in how much medicine you should take. **Over-the-counter drugs** are medicines you can buy without a prescription from the doctor. All medicines, even those on the supermarket shelves or from your doctor, can be dangerous if not taken properly.

Illegal drugs are different from prescribed drugs and far more dangerous. Prescribed or legal over-the-counter drugs are made in sterile laboratories. Trained people make sure all the ingredients are carefully measured and controlled. Illegal drugs are bought "on the street." Users usually buy them from people they don't know. They also don't know what is actually in the drugs. A mixture of "dirty" chemicals and uncontrolled drugs can kill people trying to get high.

There are four main types of drugs. **Stimulants** speed up the central nervous system and increase brain activity. Depressants, such as alcohol, slow down the central nervous system and decrease brain activity. **Hallucinogens** play with a user's mind. They change the way people see and hear things. **Analgesics** are pain-relieving drugs. They can also make a person feel warm and happy.

Stimulants
Methamphetamines

The drugs in this group are also known as *speed*, *uppers*, *meth*, *crystal meth*, and *crank*. They increase the heart rate, blood pressure, and body temperature. Methamphetamines can be swallowed, inhaled, smoked, or injected.

Many people take this type of drug when they want to stay awake for long periods of time. They think they will have more energy and be able to get more done. It gives them a quick, intense high. This makes meth highly addictive. Users want this high all the time.

But the long-term effects of this drug include mood disturbances, aggression, and **paranoia**. Paranoia causes people to feel that everyone is out to get them. It can even make users want to kill other people or themselves. Meth use also causes brain damage. The brain damage is similar to damage caused by **Alzheimer's disease**, **stroke**, and **epilepsy**.

Meth Labs

The use of methamphetamines has been growing across the country. Why? One reason is because meth is easy to make. Making meth is called "cooking." Even though many of the ingredients are common household products, mixing those products is very dangerous. It can cause explosions or release poisonous gases. Meth labs are found both in crowded neighborhoods and in rural areas throughout the nation. Sadly, many children are found living in working meth labs.

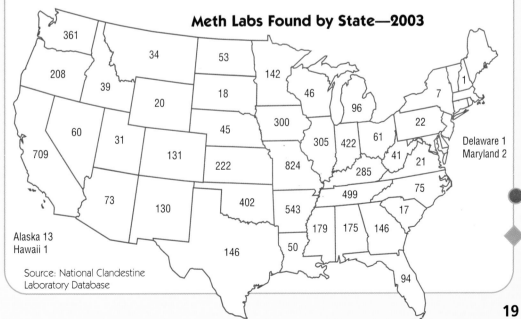

Meth Labs Found by State—2003

Alaska 13
Hawaii 1

Delaware 1
Maryland 2

Source: National Clandestine Laboratory Database

Cocaine

This white powder, also called *coke, snow*, or *blow*, comes from the coca plant, which grows in South America. When the leaf is cut and crushed, it becomes a powder that can be injected into the veins or snorted into the nose. The form of cocaine that can be smoked is called *crack*. When smoking crack, the user experiences the high in less than ten seconds. This is one reason it is so widely abused. Like so many drugs, young people think this drug is good because it makes them feel energized and excited. It gives them a quick high, but that soon wears off. This makes their brains work overtime. Even first-time users can suffer from heart attacks or **brain seizures** and die. People who use this drug often suffer from anger and violent outbursts, frustration, and **hallucinations**. Snorting the drug can also damage the inside of the nose, causing nosebleeds and constant sniffing.

Ecstasy

This drug comes in the form of a pill and is known as *E, X, XTC, Adam*, or *bean*. Drug users try this pill hoping it will make them more popular or outgoing at parties or dance clubs. Some of the side effects are teeth clenching, unusual displays of affection, chills, and sweating. But it can also be deadly. It can cause a person's body to dehydrate. It can also lead to kidney, liver, or heart failure. All of these can result in death.

A Drug That's Been Around the Block

Cocaine itself has been abused for more than 100 years. But people have eaten coca leaves for thousands of years!

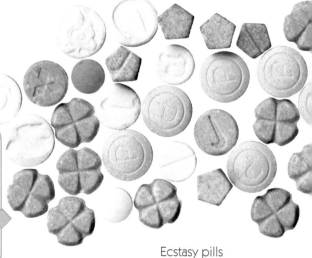

Ecstasy pills

Depressants

Tranquilizers

Tranquilizers are taken to reduce stress and relax muscles. When these are prescribed by a doctor, the patient must pay careful attention to instructions. But some people use these drugs without a doctor's prescription. To people who use these drugs illegally, they are also known as *ludes*, *downers*, and *goofballs*. When taken improperly, they can cause confusion, depression, forgetfulness, and clumsiness. Overdosing on, or taking too much or too many, tranquilizers can kill. Mixing them with other drugs or alcohol can also be deadly.

Inhalants

Inhalants are household substances that are sniffed or inhaled to give a person a dizzy or high feeling. It is similar to the feeling of being drunk. Inhalants slow breathing and heart rate. Long-term effects include headaches, nosebleeds, and permanent brain damage. Inhalants can also cause death due to lack of oxygen.

Silent Killers Lurking in Your House

These are just some of the inhalants abused by kids:

- glue
- paint
- paint thinners
- magic markers
- correction fluid
- hair spray
- air freshener
- vegetable cooking spray
- fuel canisters

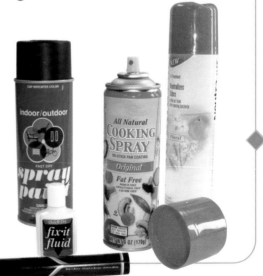

Because it involves inhaling legal, everyday household products, many kids are attracted to this high. Inhalants are the third-most abused substance among 12- to 14-year-olds in this country. But kids don't stop to think about the dangers of this pastime. Hundreds of children die each year from inhaling or sniffing gases, glues, or aerosols. Spraying aerosols down the throat can make you die instantly. If you don't die from inhaling these dangerous products, you are likely to suffer severe brain damage. Vapors from inhalants dissolve the brain's fatty tissues. This means that you could lose the ability to walk, talk, and think. Even though they are not "street drugs," inhalants are so dangerous that even one sniff can kill you!

Signs of Inhalant Abuse

- Red or runny eyes or nose
- Spots or sores around the mouth
- Unusual breath odor
- Constantly smelling shirtsleeves
- Paint or stain marks or correction fluid on clothing or skin

Hallucinogens

Marijuana

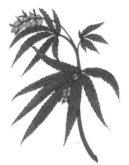

Of all the illegal drugs, marijuana is the most widely used. Its formal name is *Cannabis sativa*, but it is called *pot*, *dope*, *reefer*, *herb*, *grass*, *weed*, and even a girl's name— Mary Jane. This drug is usually rolled into a small cigarette called a *joint* or smoked through a pipe. It is a mind-altering drug. It has the power to change your view of the world around you so that you can't really be sure what you are feeling, thinking, or seeing.

People who use marijuana say they like it because it makes them feel relaxed and content. In truth, they are stepping outside reality. Their mind plays tricks on them.

Marijuana makes it hard for people to concentrate. They often lose track of time and have problems remembering and learning. It's no wonder that people who use this drug are often referred to as *stoners* or *burnouts*. They often appear to be half-asleep or just stupid.

As users become addicted to marijuana, they lose the desire to do other things. They don't want to go to school or work. They can't play sports as well as they once did. They become irresponsible and unsocial. They lose their self-esteem and confidence. And then there are real health problems to deal with. Smoking this drug causes lung damage, heart disease, and blood-circulation problems.

LSD

Also known as *acid* or *trip*, LSD changes a person's sense of space, time, and distance. Once a person takes LSD, it usually takes 12 hours to wear off. In this time, the user can have panic attacks, see scary images, or be confused and sad. LSD also causes the heart to beat faster and the blood pressure to rise.

Analgesics

Heroin

Heroin is a pain-relieving drug. But unlike legal analgesics such as codeine, morphine, and even acetometaphin (Tylenol), heroin has serious side effects. It's also very addicting. Besides the fact that it is a dangerous, powerful drug, heroin is frightening for another reason. Also known as *smack*, *junk*, or *brown sugar*, it is commonly mixed with other drugs when sold by drug dealers. Users of this drug never really know what they are getting when they inject this drug into their veins. Heroin is often linked to the spread of AIDS and **hepatitis** because drug users share the needles with which they inject themselves. If the drug itself does not kill users, something they contract from a used needle can.

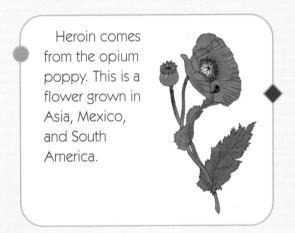

Heroin comes from the opium poppy. This is a flower grown in Asia, Mexico, and South America.

Bigger, Faster, Stronger: Drugs in Sports

Not all people use drugs just to get the high. Some people choose to use drugs because they want to do better in sports. They care so much about winning that they don't care about their own health or the welfare of others. Many times, athletes become frustrated that they cannot run faster, kick harder, or lift more. They look for something that will help them be stronger or faster than anyone else. Unfortunately, some athletes and coaches turn to drugs for help.

The use of drugs to make a person perform better in sports is called *doping*. Some popular drugs used in sports are steroids, androstenedione, and ephedrine. All of these are banned by at least some athletic organizations. That means the drugs are not allowed in those organized sports. For this reason, athletes must lie and cheat if they want to take the drugs.

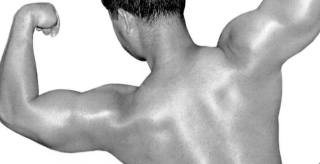

Steroids

Anabolic steroids are **hormones** that develop bigger muscles and increase muscle tissue in the human body. Also known as *roids* or *juice*, steroids are similar to the male hormone called **testosterone**. Steroids are found naturally in the body. But some athletes take extra steroids to become bigger and stronger. Surveys show that young people are using steroids more often.

When you pump extra things into your body that are not meant to be there naturally—like extra testosterone—side effects occur. Heart disease, liver damage, cancer, **urinary** and **bowel** problems, strokes, and blood clots are all side effects of taking steroids. They are also all life-threatening. Less dangerous side effects are the possibility of going bald and getting **acne**. Steroids make boys more feminine and girls more masculine. They can also make it impossible for the user to have children, even later in life. And for kids and teens, steroids make you permanently stop growing. Steroid users also suffer from emotional side effects. These include severe mood swings, violent anger, depression, and thoughts of suicide.

Out of Control

It is so common for steroid users to become aggressive and easily angered that the term "roid rage" has been created.

Androstenedione

Androstenedione, also known as *andro*, is like steroids. It doesn't cause muscle growth on its own. But once in the body, it is changed into testosterone. Then it works just like steroids to increase muscle mass. Like steroids, andro's side effects include cancer, stroke, and increased risk of heart disease. The use of androstendione with young people also causes growth to be halted. Like steroids, androstendione is banned by such organizations as the National Collegiate Athletics Association (NCAA), the National Football League (NFL), and the International Olympic Committee.

Ephedrine

Ephedrine is a drug also known as *ephedra* or *ma huang*. Like other stimulants, these pills speed up your nervous system and increase **metabolism**, which burns fat. Some athletes take ephedrine because they want to lose weight, improve concentration, and perform better. However, research has not shown that ephedrine makes a person stronger, quicker, or able to work out longer.

What does ephedrine do? Ephedrine has many side effects. It increases the heart rate and makes the blood pressure rise. If too much is taken, it can cause a person to have a heart attack. It also causes dizziness and headaches. Strokes are other possible effects. It is especially dangerous to use ephedrine with caffeine, which is found in soft drinks and energy drinks.

Ephedrine is banned in the Olympics and in college sports. It is also banned in the NFL.

A Tragic Lesson

People in the sports world took a closer look at ephedrine after the death of a young pitcher from the Baltimore Orioles named Steve Bechler in 2003. An examination showed that the use of ephedrine played a part in his death from heatstroke. He was only 23 years old.

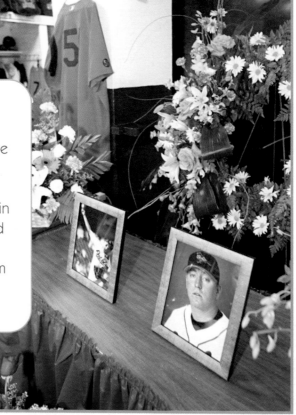

Can't Get Enough
Addiction

If you look up the word *addict* in the dictionary, you will find a description of someone who cannot control his or her own behavior. When people become addicted to something, they no longer have the power to get away from it or say no to it. Very few addicts are able to stop taking drugs without professional help. Addiction—whether it is to alcohol, drugs, or even something else like gambling—is a disease. And like all diseases, if it is not treated, it will continue to spread, causing more and more damage. Addicts become so sick that they need their drug to feel "normal." But each time they take a drug or drink alcohol, the addiction worsens.

While addiction is not a choice, choosing to experiment with drugs and alcohol is. The best way to avoid addiction is to avoid the behavior. When you say, "No!", harmful things can't hurt you.

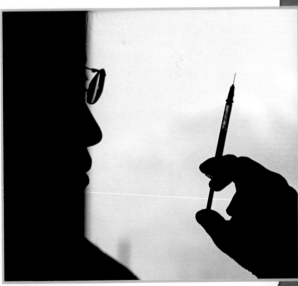

Drug Abuse vs. Drug Addiction

What's the difference? When you are sick and your doctor prescribes a drug, he or she describes how you should use it. For example, your prescription might say, "One pill every six hours." If you take more than that, you are abusing the drug. It is important to follow the instructions because only the doctor knows exactly how much of the medicine you need to get well. If you take too little, your body doesn't get the help it needs. If you take too much, your body can get confused. It may stop working to get well. Then, your body may start sending messages to your brain that say, "I can't get well by myself. I need more medicine . . . and more . . . and more."

Why does this happen? It's because of something called **neurotransmitters**. Here's how neurotransmitters work.

Let's say your teacher tells you that you just earned an A and that you are one of the smartest students she has ever had. Wouldn't that be great? Obviously, this would make you very happy. Every time something good happens, your brain releases neurotransmitters. These chemicals release pleasant messages to your brain, making you feel happy.

But when people use drugs, their brains begin to rely on drugs to get those pleasure messages. Everything begins to get jumbled up inside their minds. Soon, because they have been taking drugs, their brains tell the neurotransmitters to slow down. Can you guess what happens next? The drug abusers become depressed and have less energy. Then they take even more drugs to feel better. Each time they take more medication or drugs, their feeling of happiness lasts a

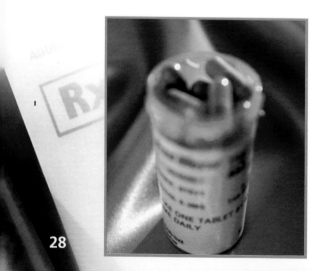

shorter amount of time. Soon, they move from being drug abusers to drug addicts.

Who, Me? No Way!

The truth is, anyone can become addicted to drugs, tobacco, or alcohol. Scientists have determined that **heredity** plays a big part in how and why people become addicted. This means that if a family member has an addiction problem, you are more likely to have one too. While there are a number of reasons a person would be willing to try drugs in the first place (to be cool, to be a rebel, to make friends, to stop feelings of depression or anger), some people may be more likely to become addicts than others. This is why some kids will try smoking and then decide they don't like it and never smoke again, and other kids will try it and get hooked.

How Do You Know If Your Friend or Family Member Is Using Drugs?

You can't count on addicts. They break promises, do not show up for appointments, and don't return phone calls. Drug addicts have a difficult time keeping jobs, friends, and family members. Because they are so worried about how they will get their next bottle of alcohol or pill, addicts are unable to focus on your wants and needs.

When your friend or family member stops caring about school, friends, or family, it could be a sign of drug use. This could mean being late for work or school, or not doing a job or homework properly. Of course, these behaviors can be signs of other problems going on in the person's life. But when the person you care about seems to be grumpy or depressed much of the time, doesn't want to hang out or talk, and asks to be left alone, something is probably wrong. When there is a sudden change in the person's appearance, it can mean the addiction to the drugs or alcohol is taking over. Changes can be weight loss, shaking, coughing, red eyes, or clumsiness. Talk to your friend or loved one and try to find out what is going on.

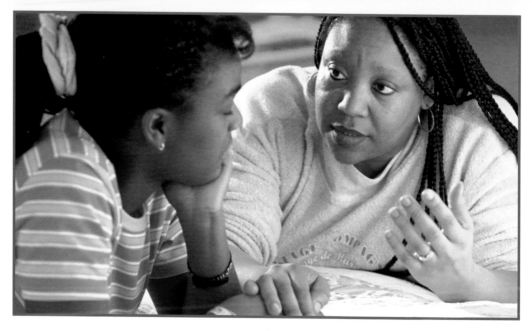

What You Can Do

Maybe your friend or family member won't talk to you. Addicts usually don't admit or understand how bad their problems are. When they lose their jobs, crash a car, or have fights with friends, they blame other things or people. This is part of their sickness. Because they are scared, they are unable to ask for help. The whole situation may seem hopeless, but there are things you can do to help.

First, find an adult you can talk to. A teacher, school counselor, coach, minister, or rabbi can be very helpful. They will know who to contact and how to find professional help for your friend or family member. It is important to find an adult who understands the problem and can keep you safe while help is sought. Many times addicts become frightened that their alcohol or drugs will be taken away from them. They can become angry—even violent. For this reason, you need to have a teacher, counselor, or doctor do the talking. If you are unable to find an adult you can trust, there are organizations you can call. You can talk to a trained professional—a person who talks to family members and friends of addicts all the time. These professionals will be able to answer questions and tell you what you should do.

Organizations That Can Help

- **Alcohol and Other Drug Information for Teens** (www.child.net/drugalc.htm)

  The National Children's Coalition offers facts about drugs and alcohol for teens and kids, provides recovery group therapy, and serves as a resource center.

- **Alcoholics Anonymous** (www.alcoholics-anonymous.org)

  This is a national organization that can answer questions and provide help for you and your family members. Because they want you to reach out for help, you can talk to them without worrying about them telling anyone else.

- **American Council for Drug Education** (www.acde.org)

  This organization provides education about drugs and how families are affected by addictions. They serve as a resource center for treatment and can answer questions.

- **National Substance Abuse Help Line** (www.drughelp.org)

  People can access this Web site or call 1-800-662-HELP to get answers and to speak to someone who understands everything they are feeling.

- **Students Against Destructive Decisions** (www.sadd.org)

  This leadership group for kids discusses how to prevent underage drinking, other drug use, and impaired driving.

Excuses, Excuses
Myths About Alcohol, Tobacco, and Drugs

So, after reading all of the facts, it has to make you wonder—why would anyone in the world abuse drugs or alcohol or use tobacco? Here are some of the excuses you might hear.

"Everyone Is Doing It!"

No. Not everyone is doing it. The majority of people stay away from drugs, tobacco, and alcohol because they understand how dangerous it is for their health and for the people around them. People involved with drugs are more likely to be victims of crime or involved in criminal activity than people who are not drug users. In other words, when you hang around drugs, you are more likely to be in dangerous places or with dangerous people. If *everyone* around you is doing these things, you need to find new friends. These are not people who care about you or will be able to help you in times of trouble.

"It Makes Me More Relaxed!"

Certain drugs or alcohol slow down the way you think. They make you think and react more slowly and kill brain cells. While you may *feel* relaxed, the truth is your brain and body are not working correctly.

"It Makes Me More Creative!"

Because drugs affect the way you think and feel, it only appears you are more creative. In reality, you are anything but creative. You cannot think clearly, you cannot speak clearly, and you are endangering your brain and body. This is not creativity. This is called *self-destruction*.

"Drugs Help Me!"

Initially, people who use tobacco, alcohol, or drugs say that these substances help them. They say they feel more confident and secure when they are drinking, smoking, or high. They have less pain or believe they are stronger. However, once addicted, the addicts' bodies want and need more and more of the substance. Their bodies and brains then begin to break down. To say alcohol, tobacco, or drugs help anyone is far from the truth.

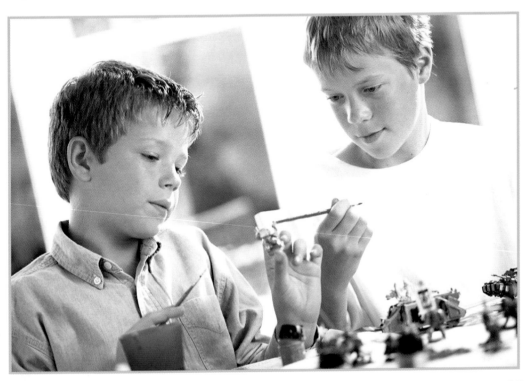

Many people believe the myth that "Drugs aren't bad if you can control them." You can't control drugs. The truth is that as your body becomes addicted to the drugs, the drugs begin to control you. This is also true when you smoke and drink. Remember, this is your life and you should always be in control.

And how do drugs help you create a future? Imagine that you have a friend or an older brother who has begun using drugs. For one reason or another, your brother or friend has asked you to hold a little bag of marijuana for a couple of days. You say, "Hey, I don't like this stuff," but your brother or friend tells you, "It's just for a couple of days. Just do it for me this one time and I won't ever ask you again." You might be tempted, but if you are caught holding on to that little bag of drugs, you could get into a lot of trouble. You could even be arrested. And, you're not helping your friend or your brother. You are making it harder for him to admit his problem and get help.

What's the Truth?

Think about your life and your future. When you dream, what do you dream about? Becoming a famous athlete? A teacher? A marine biologist who gets to work with dolphins and whales? Or perhaps a scientist, creating new ways to travel to other planets? Maybe you wish you could one day be a great guitar player, a violinist, or an amazing artist. All of these things are just dreams if you become involved with drugs, including tobacco and alcohol. One of the worst things about drugs is that the more you use them, the fewer dreams you have. Drugs kill everything— hopes, dreams, friendships, health, and happiness.

Only you are in charge of your own future. You must learn to stand up for yourself and be ready to live out your own dreams. If someone is pushing you to try drugs, cigarettes, or alcohol, tell them, "No!" If this person doesn't listen, talk to an adult about how to handle him or her. He or she is certainly not

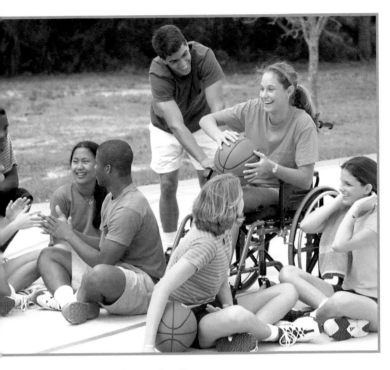

When you watch the Olympics and see athletes win medals or break world records, remember that they are living their dreams. When you read a great book, know that the author had dreams and now writes about those dreams. Presidents become presidents because they had dreams of greatness. Inventors invent and scientists create because they all had dreams. And all of these people studied and worked to achieve their dreams.

Everything you do in life will impact your future. To have the future you want, you have to make good decisions that will help you move toward that future. Put yourself on the right track. Your dreams can come true!

your friend and doesn't care about your future.

When you are faced with a difficult problem, something scary or unpleasant, don't try to hide from it by taking drugs. Speaking about things that bother or upset you is the smartest and safest thing to do. Find an adult or someone you trust to talk to. Drugs can't help you get better grades, make more friends, or have a happier life. Talking about real feelings to real people is the only way to figure out your problems.

Internet Connections and Related Readings for *Alcohol, Tobacco, and Drugs*

American Council for Drug Education (www.acde.org/youth/)

Find out all about drugs and how they affect your body. Visit an art gallery where kids from a drug treatment center have explored art as part of their therapy. Then test your smarts with a "Got the smarts?" knowledge quiz about drugs and what they can do to you.

Campaign for Tobacco-Free Kids (www. tobaccofreekids.org)

Read the latest news and headlines about tobacco, especially as they relate to kids. Look up research and facts about tobacco use. Find out how you can become involved in helping other kids say no to tobacco. Browse the Tobacco Ad Gallery to see full images of print ads from different tobacco companies, even ads from different countries.

Partnership for a Drug-Free America (www.drugfreeamerica.org)

Read about any type of drug and learn why that drug is harmful to you. Explore stories of young people whose lives were forever changed by drugs. Get answers to questions you may have, such as how to tell if a friend has a drug problem or how to tell if your own drug or alcohol use is out of control. The Campaign Viewer allows you to access the PDFA's latest television, radio, and print messages. Learn more about some of your favorite musicians and sports figures and why they stay drug-free.

Up and Down the Mountain: Helping Children Cope with Parental Alcoholism by Pamela Leib Higgins. Jenny wonders if her father, an alcoholic, will attend her 6th grade graduation. New Horizons Press, 2002. [RL 4, IL 2–5] (EA3404901 PB)

Glossary

acne (AK nee) bumps and blemishes that occur on the skin

addicted (uhd DIKT uhd) dependent on a harmful drug

AIDS (aydz) a disease of the **immune system** caused by infection with the HIV virus. There is no cure for AIDS. (see separate entry)

alcohol (AL kuh hahl) a liquid that is a **depressant** when consumed by a person (see separate entry)

alcohol poisoning (AL kuh hahl POY zuhn ing) the state of drinking too much **alcohol** in too short a time, which can cause loss of **consciousness** and death (see separate entries)

alcoholics (al kuh HAHL iks) people who are **addicted** to drinking **alcohol** (see separate entries)

alveoli (al vee OH lee) tiny, thin-walled air sacs found in the **lungs** (see separate entry)

Alzheimer's disease (AHLZ heyem erz diz EEZ) a disease that affects the brain, causing confusion that continually becomes worse

analgesics (an uhl JEE ziks) drugs that relieve pain

bowel (BOW uhl) relating to the intestines, part of the digestive system

brain seizures (brayn SEE zherz) sudden attacks on the brain that can cause a **coma** or death (see separate entry)

bronchial tubes (BRAHN kee uhl toobz) tubular passages that bring air to and from the **lungs** (see separate entry)

cancer (KAN ser) growth caused when cells multiply uncontrollably, destroying healthy tissue

carbon dioxide (KAR buhn deye AWK seyed) a gas breathed out by humans

central nervous system (SEN truhl NERV uhs SIS tuhm) the part of the body that includes the brain and the spinal cord and controls most functions of the body and mind

cigarettes (sig uh RETS) rolls of shredded **tobacco** leaves in a thin paper used for smoking (see separate entry)

coma (KOH muh) long, deep state of being unable to see, hear, or sense what is going on around oneself

consciousness (KAHN shuhs nes) the state of being awake and aware of what is going on around oneself

depressant (duh PRES uhnt) drug that causes the brain to slow down

doping (DOHP ing) the use of drugs to enhance performance in athletics

drugs (druhgz) substances that cause changes in behavior, the way a person feels, and the way a person sees the world

epilepsy (ep uh LEP see) disease that causes sudden loss of **consciousness** and often jerking muscle spasms (see separate entry)

hallucinations (huhl loo suh NAY shunz) instances where people think they see or hear things that aren't really there

hallucinogens (huhl loo SIN uh jenz) drugs that cause people to see or hear things that aren't really there

hangover (HANG oh ver) the symptoms of headache, **vomiting**, thirst, and sickness that result from drinking too much **alcohol** (see separate entries)

hepatitis (hep uh TEYE tuhs) disease in which the liver, an organ necessary for humans to live, becomes inflamed

herbs (erbz) plants that can be used to make medications or for good health

heredity (huh RED uh tee) the passing of genetic factors, such as the color of hair or eyes, from one generation in a family to the next

hormones (HOR mohnz) special chemicals a person's body makes to help it do certain things, such as build muscles or mature

immune system (im MYOON SIS tuhm) body system that creates a defense against foreign substances

intoxicated (in TAWKS uh kay tuhd) having drunk too much **alcohol** (see separate entry)

lethal (LEE thuhl) causing or able to cause death

lungs (luhngz) two spongy, saclike organs located in the chest that inflate and enable **oxygen** to get to the heart (see separate entry)

market (MAR ket) to use advertising to attract buyers to a product for sale

metabolism (muh TAB uh lizm) the fat-burning mechanism that allows people to burn calories and stay trim

neurotransmitters (new roh TRANS mit terz) chemicals in the brain that carry messages to other parts of the body about how the person feels

nicotine (NIK uh teen) poisonous substance found in **tobacco** products (see separate entry)

over-the-counter drugs (OH ver *the* KOWNT er druhgz) drugs sold directly to the public without a doctor's prescription

oxygen (AWK suh juhn) a gas that humans breathe in that is necessary for life

paranoia (pair uh NOY uh) mental disorder in which people believe other people or things are out to get them

prescription drugs (pruh SKRIP shuhn druhgz) drugs that can only be obtained through doctors' orders

smokeless tobacco (SMOHK les tuh BAK koh) **tobacco** that is not smoked but put between the gums and lips and sucked on (see separate entry)

stimulants (STIM yoo luhnts) drugs that produce a temporary increase in the activity of a body organ or part

stroke (strohk) sudden blockage of or bursting of a blood vessel in the brain, which results in loss of **consciousness**, partial loss of movement, or loss of speech (see separate entry)

surgeon general (SER juhn JEN uh ruhl) the chief medical officer in the United States Public Health Service

testosterone (tes TAHS tuhr ohn) a male **hormone** produced in the body (see separate entry)

tobacco (tuh BAK koh) any of the products made from the leaves of the tobacco plant, such as cigarettes

urinary (YOO ri nair ee) relating to urine, liquid waste product, or the organs that form and get rid of urine

vomiting (VAHM uht ing) expelling the contents of the stomach through the mouth as a result of involuntary spasms of the stomach muscles

Index